How to lose weight

effortlessly

Vienela Sas

Important ideas explained for everyone to understand

CONTENTS

Author's note:

I apologize in advance because my English is not very good. I know you will understand me, however, as I have been understood by all the people I have been talking to for four years, since I have lived in Scotland.
I consider that, beyond grammatical rules or sometimes wrongly chosen words, the message that the book conveys is important. I wish with all my heart that I can help you lose weight healthily, that you can move freely and love yourself as you deserve.
I want you to look at this book as a dialogue you have with a trusted friend who understands and supports you. I can do this for you beyond the book, if you feel the need to talk to someone who knows exactly what you are going through.
We will travel this difficult road together, and in the end we will enjoy the results together.
I can't afford to ask you to trust me completely. I just invite you to try the methods I recommend in the book.

These are simple things that anyone can do if they are motivated enough. We will work together on motivation, because it is the most important engine.

Probably many of the tips are already known to you, but you haven't tested them in the long run so far.

It's time to take courage and work on your own health and happiness.

I will be with you throughout the process you will go through. I will be the shoulder to lean on when you feel you are losing your motivation, when you want to give up, when you think you can't complete the "mission".

Let's start!

How to lose weight
fast and healthy without effort?

I know, you asked yourself this question every day and tried all the diets and recipes that got in your way on the internet, in books or when talking to other people, friends or even strangers.

You have already noticed that nothing has had a long-term effect. Even if you managed to lose weight for a while, the moment you finished the diet you gained weight again. You have been hungry many times, hoping that you will be able to lose weight.

Sometimes you paid too much money for some big lies. The world is full of charlatans who do not care about people's health and feelings. They just want to get rich by taking advantage of man's naivete or hot desire to solve a certain problem he is facing.

You would like to wear certain clothes and they do not fit you, and that contributes to the bad mood you sometimes have. Whether the clothing manufacturers make certain models only for the weak, or for example you consider that a very short skirt does not fit a plump woman, the problem exists and affects your psyche.

The problem has often arisen that movies and TV shows contribute to the idea that only weak people are beautiful. As wrong as the idea is, it does so much harm to ordinary people who do not have the perfect body.

We live in a wrongly constructed world, where a person's value is given by her beauty.

You are probably jealous of skinny girls who can eat anything without fear of gaining weight. You don't feel good about yourself and you don't want to look in the mirror anymore.

I do not judge you. I know all this because I once gained a few extra pounds and I suffered because the boys were looking for skinny girls.

This is what happens in Romania, my native country, where men like "plank" women, as we Romanians say, "string, no tits, no ass".

I already know that this is wrong, because it makes girls not trust themselves and, often, they try wrong methods to lose weight fast.

I make a parenthesis to tell you what happened to me when I arrived in Scotland. I was very thin at the time, I weighed about 50 kg (110.2 pounds (lbs)) at 1.70 m (5.6 feet). I was at work with a colleague, also Romanian. She was joking with a Scottish man on a sensual subject.

At one point, the man told her that she was too thin, that he liked chubby girls. I looked better at my colleague.
She weighed about 8 kg more than me. I laughed when I imagined what the Scotsman thought of me, if he considered her weak. In his eyes, I was probably long dead.
But let's get back to our topic. Many years ago, I also suffered because I felt bad when I went to the beach. I could see my cellulite and my body was too big next to other women. I felt inhibited every time I stayed in a swimsuit.
If I ate with other people, I had the impression that everyone was laughing at me because I ate too much. I was hungry and I wanted to eat all kinds of food, but I was trying to refrain from becoming the target of the ironies of those around me.
I was only about 8-10 kilograms more than I should have been and I felt horrible. I realize how women / girls who weigh more weight feel. I understand them perfectly, because I have lived all this and much more.
Believe it or not, I was once jealous even of my sister, who had a flat stomach and strong arms. It's not a normal feeling for a human being.

Let me help you lose weight

I'm going to tell you things that you may have heard many times before, though not in this form. I will support you in your effort to lose weight (not very) fast and at the same time healthy.

You just have to believe me when I tell you that there is no miracle recipe to do this for you. Your will, your desire to look good and be healthy - this is the best medicine to lose weight.

When she was 65, my mother suffered a stroke that immobilized her in bed. She was paralyzed and depended on others for a living. She always said to me: Vienela, you stay on the internet all day long. You look there, maybe you can find a medicine that I can take to heal myself and get out of bed. Unfortunately, there are no drugs that work wonders.

Ask yourself how much you want to have a slim body, to be able to move freely, to run, to swim, to wear the clothes you like. Look in the mirror and tell yourself if you like what you see. Are you happy with the way you look? Would you like to get rid of the belly that you consider to be too big? Do you want to have thinner legs? Have beautiful arms and slim waist?

Mental training

The biggest mistake a person who wants to lose weight can make is to start directly by doing too much gymnastics or starving. Do not do this! You will quickly run out and you will lose the desire to try again.

You must first mentally prepare for what is to come. How to do that? Here are some ways to prepare your mind, get used to the idea that you will work to have a leaner and healthier body:

1. Get some routine medical tests to make sure you're healthy. Sometimes people gain weight because of health problems. If you feel good physically, it does not necessarily mean that you are healthy. There are certain diseases that are hidden in the body. They can be detected on routine medical tests. If everything is ok in terms of physical health, you can move on to the next level.

2. Prepare a journal where to write down what you want to tick. On amazon, at my author profile, (Vienela Sas) you will find the most suitable diary, because it is made in such a way as to be in accordance with this book, with my advice in it.

Write down in your diary everything you like and don't like about yourself. I will give you some examples: you like that you have beautiful eyes, you dance very well, you have a charming smile, your hair shines in wonderful colors, your skin is fine, velvety, you are intelligent, you have a good soul, you have a cheerful nature and you are used to laughing a lot etc.

Write about what you don't like about yourself: you can't wear high-heeled sandals, your face is too round, with puffy cheeks, you can't hide the fact that you have a belly fat, you are inhibited in the presence of other women, etc.

Write down the reasons why you want to lose so much weight. Write as honestly as you can, to realize how much you are affected by the fact that you do not have the dream figure and to have a permanent desire to fight to achieve your goal.

Write down in your journal absolutely all the progress and efforts you make to reach the target. It doesn't matter if it's just the fact that you gave up a candy today. Make a note of this in your journal. You will notice after a while that every candy you gave up contributed to the fight you are fighting against the extra pounds.

3. You start by setting a target: how many kilograms do you want to lose and for how long? Don't set goals you know you can't reach. You start with small steps. For example, determine that you want to lose 3 kg in 30 days.

4. Take pictures every day, preferably dressed in the same clothes. They will be the clearest proof that your work has paid off and that you have really managed to lose weight.

5. Write down on paper several small objectives that you want to reach and stick them around the house, in the visible places. They can be daily, weekly, monthly, etc. goals.

For example, you can write on a note that you will not open the fridge more than five times today. Stick the note on the fridge.

Or write on a note that this week you want to walk 15 minutes every day, no matter what the weather will be like. Stick the note on the door.

Or that this month you want to dance at least ten times at home on a certain song. Stick the ticket on the TV or computer screen.

6. Form a morning routine that contributes to your well-being and your desire to lose weight. Take a shower every morning, ventilate the house

well and dress nicely even if you are not going anywhere. You will see that you start your day with a smile on your face and with the conviction that you can do whatever you want.

Don't be embarrassed or afraid of mistakes. You are human and it is natural to have moments when you feel that you no longer want to do a certain thing. It is natural to sometimes feel tired, disappointed or angry. We all have such moments. You will probably have days when you want to stop, to give up any attempt to fight the extra pounds.

I advise you not to give in to impulse. It will pass if you fight him. Instead of lying on the couch crying or swearing, get dressed and get out of the house. Take a walk and eat an ice cream. Listen to music and take pictures of the nature around you.

You may think I'm cruel or bad at what I say, but I recommend you read books and documentaries about the sufferings of those who were prisoners in Nazi concentration camps. Read about children in Africa and all their suffering. Ryan Hreljac's story will impress you to tears and show you another face of the world. The fight you are going through will not seem so hard anymore.

As you already know, food is the most important factor. Try to reduce portions of food. I won't tell you to eat a lettuce leaf at lunch, because it's absurd.

I don't want to make you suffer or give up before you succeed. I just ask you to reduce a little of the portion you prepared. As little as you want, so that you can note in the diary that you have made this effort.

For example, if you usually eat two buns at a meal, set for the first week to eat only one bun and three-quarters of the second. No matter how good the food on the plate, it doesn't eat absolutely everything. Leave at least one tablespoon of food on the plate. It will be your way of fighting, of proving that you can do everything you set out to do.

Really realistic goals are the ones that will help you fulfill your dream.

Never miss breakfast. It is the most important meal of the day and I will explain immediately why. If you eat healthy and full in the morning, you no longer feel the need to nibble various until noon. I have for you at the end of the book some recipes for a healthy breakfast.

They will help you feel full without eating too much. Arrange the food nicely on the plate and take pictures. You will see, over time, that your portions of food will be smaller and smaller. You will have fun remembering how much food you put on the plate.

It is said by the elders that in the morning you should eat like a king, at noon like a prince, and in the evening like a beggar. This means that you need to eat well in the morning, enough at noon and very little in the evening.
At dinner, avoid foods that make you fat or that your stomach finds difficult to digest. Do not eat pork, eggs, bread, pasta, pizza in the evening and especially do not order fast food.
Instead, choose vegetables, fruits, possibly fish or a little chicken or beef.
Ideally, each meal you eat should contain a little of what matters: meat, vegetables, dairy and grains. Italians are world famous for eating healthy: a portion of pasta with meat that includes bell peppers and onions, and sprinkle with grated cheese on top, is a perfectly healthy and filling meal.

It is very important to eat fruit. The body needs energy, and fruits can give you the energy you need. In addition, they are perfect for fast digestion.

Avoid eating between meals, especially fast food or sweets such as chocolate or pastries.

Are the above tips enough to help you lose weight fast and healthy?

No, it's definitely not enough to be careful about food. In order to lose weight you have to do other things, which I will tell you about immediately.

I know, it's very hard to get out of your comfort zone, change your routine and do things you haven't done in a long time, but that's the only way you can lose weight healthily.

You have to understand that in the first days after you start reducing your food portions, you will be hungry. You will have the feeling that you must nibble on something, that you are on the verge of fainting from hunger. Refrain. It's just a momentary sensation. Eat an apple or look for an activity that will distract you.

It won't be long and you will forget how hungry you were a few minutes ago. In fact, your stomach does not suffer if you give it less food, on the contrary.

Your stomach will make less effort trying to digest what you gave it, and this will make you more active, able to move more freely, feel better physically and mentally. I'm sure you will succeed! Don't let your own brain fool you that you can't stay without eating like you used to.

Make as much movement as possible. It is extremely important not to sit on a chair or sofa after eating, whether it is breakfast, lunch or dinner. This is one of the main reasons why people gain weight.

Get up, wash the dishes, sweep the kitchen, tidy the house. If you're not the kind of housewife who works all day to keep the house gleaming (welcome to the group; I'm not either), go for a short walk around the neighborhood. Walk at least 1-2 kilometers (at least a mile, if you live in the UK).

You can also exercise at home, but it is preferable to go for a walk, breathe fresh air and have time to meditate on everything you have achieved so far.

If you are at work, look for reasons to move from your chair: go to the bathroom, go out to smoke a cigarette, go to the office next door to talk to a colleague, etc.

Make it a habit to dance every day. Whenever you have the opportunity, dress nicely, sit in front of the mirror and dance. You will notice how beautiful you are, how graceful you move and how good you would look if you weighed a few kilograms. This will motivate you to work harder to reach the result you are aiming for.

Dancing is a great way to exercise, avoid sedentary lifestyles and strengthen your muscles. In addition, when you dance, your mood changes. You feel happier, stronger, more alive, more motivated.

You may have a big surprise after a while, as my sister had when she was trying to lose weight by dancing a lot. Well, although she looked much slimmer, every time she weighed herself, her weight was about the same.

You know why? Because instead of fat, muscles developed that she hadn't used much before. And muscle is heavier than fat, isn't it?

My sister continued to dance and strengthen her muscles. Her body took on a beautiful shape. Her waist was clear, her legs were well contoured, and her belly was getting flatter. And all this just because she made time to dance for at least half an hour every day, in a few rounds.

Avoid commercial juices and carbonated drinks. All contain sugar and / or various fattening sweeteners. Choose better to make your own juices from well-ripened fruit. Put a little lemon juice in the fresh juice. Drink lemonade in which you put only a little honey. Drink as much water as you can.

Avoid pork, chicken skin (which contains a lot of fat) and sweets. Although some studies show that chicken skin is an unsaturated fat, so a healthy food, I advise you to avoid it and eat chicken breast instead.

Of course, you can eat from time to time, if chicken skin is among your favorite foods, but please do not overdo it. Everything that is in excess harms the human body, whether we are talking about seemingly good things or bad things.

If you like animals, maybe it's time to get a dog. It will motivate you to leave the house every day, to make a lot of exercise and, in addition, it will love you as you are, without judging you or laughing at you. For your pet, the notion of bullying does not exist.

I am the best example I can give you. A few years ago I was blogging full time. I would wake up in the morning, have a coffee and start writing. I sat at my desk until noon, without moving. During this time I drink a lot of coffee and smoke cigarette after cigarette.

My office was always full of chocolate, croissants, breadcrumbs, biscuits, soft drinks (usually Fanta or Coca-Cola) and other such snacks.

At noon I slept for an hour, then returned to my desk to do my job as a blogger. I sat in the chair until late in the evening, during which time I ate everything I could find on the desk, without measure and without control. I was always pale, tired, lifeless, stressed and nervous.

Then I adopted a dog. I found him on the street. It was a four-month-old puppy, hungry and scared. He changed my life. Thanks to him, I've been out of the house for six years at least twice a day. I walk, I laugh a lot, I have fun and I see life in pink.

Don't starve yourself in any way. When you are hungry, morale goes down to earth, and the body functions according to other parameters. You lose your energy and zest for life, your motivation to fight decreases. Don't starve.

Reducing the portion of food and not eating are two totally different things. If you stay without food for too long, you may even get sick. If you want to lose weight and stay healthy at the same time, you just have to follow the right steps, as described here.

One of the sayings I follow in life says: Eat to live, do not live to eat (in other words, eat only enough to survive and work, do not make eating a purpose in life).

Believe me when I tell you that there are no miraculous recipes. The secret is to have the will to re-educate yourself to lead an active and healthy life. To really want to prove that you can keep the situation under control, that you can take your life into your own hands and decide what to do with it.

If you need moral support, I can stand by you in the race you start. Leave me a message and we'll talk.

This is how I think your days should look like

I won't tell you what time to wake up, but the sooner you do it, the better it will be for you.

I won't even tell you what to do during the day. You know best what your current activities are. I just want you to take the time to work on our mission, because I feel directly involved in your effort to lose weight.

You probably know that in no field does success come overnight without effort. However, I want your path to a pleasant figure and a healthy body to be as smooth and easy to cross.

It is not absolutely necessary to follow the steps in the order in which I placed them here. The important thing is not to skip the stages, not to let the day go by until you tick everything on this list.

Remember that the first days are always the hardest, because you will probably have to give up certain habits, some inappropriate habits, eating too much, living a sedentary life and so on.

I am already smiling imagining what happiness will embrace you when you reach the desired weight, when you will be able to wear the clothes you like, when you will be able to look at yourself in the mirror with pride, knowing that you have overcome all your fears and that you have fallen all barriers.

1. Take a shower, perfume yourself and style your hair.
2. Dress nicely even if you know you're not going anywhere and no one is coming to visit.
3. Ventilate the house. Fresh air will awaken your zest for life and help you focus better.
4. Have breakfast. In the next chapter you will find some recipe ideas for breakfast. Use them and, why not ?, invent others.
5. Walk immediately after eating.
6. Prepare at least one note in which to write down something useful in your fight with extra pounds. Stick it somewhere in the house, in plain sight.
7. Listen to music and dance. Music gives you a feeling of well-being, and dancing helps you strengthen your muscles and eliminate excess fat.
8. Take a picture dressed in the clothes from the first day of your fight, the ones that will show you the best results you have.

9. Every week reduce a little of the portion of food. Don't forget to leave a little on your plate, even if you still feel hungry. It is a momentary sensation, a revolt of the brain.

10. After absolutely every meal of the day move. Take a walk, swim, ride a bike, tidy up the house or anything else you can and want to do. It is important not to sit on a chair, sofa or bed after you have finished eating.

11. Try to eat at the same hours every day.

12. Fruits and vegetables should not be missing from your diet.

13. Be as active as possible during the day. Any little extra exercise you do compared to your regular program contributes to weight loss.

14. Use a pedometer to keep track of how many steps you take. You will see that from one day to the next you will take more steps and you will get less and less tired.

15. Under no circumstances do you starve or exhaust yourself with exercise. Keep energy for tomorrow, because otherwise you will lose your motivation, you will feel the need to lie in bed and all your efforts so far will be in vain. Of course, in the first days you might go through all this, until you form a program and until you start to know

your body and your strengths again. It is no problem if in the first days you will take another break and rest to regain your strength.

16. Do not keep in your house food that is harmful to you, because you will be tempted to eat it.

17. Eat slowly, without haste, and get up from the table before you feel that your stomach is very full.

18. Give up alcohol. Beer, in particular, contributes decisively to gaining extra pounds, but other alcoholic beverages do you no good either.

19. Learn to read the labels of the products you buy to avoid those that contain too much salt, too many sweeteners, too many calories.

20. NEVER eat after 9 pm and do not fall asleep after midnight, but before.

21. Write daily in your journal the progress you have made. No matter how small they may seem to you, they are actually your success, small steps that lead you to the best end result. There is your work, your daily effort, your desire to have a better life.

The diary we created will help you keep track of everything you need to lose weight effortlessly.

22. If possible, find someone who has the same problem, to go this route together. Any problem is easier to solve in two. It is not easy to lose weight, but neither is it impossible.

I can support you virtually, if you want to get in touch on the internet. If you live in West Lothian, Scotland, I can support you physically, in case you want to walk together once a week. I would be more than happy to do this for you.

Recipes for a healthy breakfast and the right foods

Remember that breakfast is the most important meal of the day. The food you eat in the morning helps you stay healthy and full of life.

But more than that, it helps you have enough energy for the whole day. Other benefits: avoid digestion problems and get rid of the need to eat too much between meals and especially in the evening.

Did you know that people who skip breakfast are more prone to obesity? They are also more susceptible to cardiovascular disease. A healthy life starts with a healthy breakfast. The human body consumes resources even at night, that is, when you sleep. That is why it is important to eat enough in the morning and preferably before drinking coffee.

Breakfast is a very important meal - it can either make or break your day. You need to make sure that breakfast contains all the necessary foods. From them the body can extract the nutrients it needs to function perfectly. For this reason, the first meal of the day must be healthy, tasty and nutritious at the same time.

Therefore, breakfast should contain carbohydrates, fats and proteins. When choosing the products to eat in the morning, you need to consider a few factors:

-age
-gender
-activities during the day
-but especially the state of health

Here is a small list of ingredients from which you can prepare a quick, rich, healthy and good-looking breakfast. Don't miss roasted bread, soft boiled egg, tomatoes, cucumbers and dried fruits. Also, don't forget butter, honey, milk, tea, fresh fruit, cucumbers, pumpkin seeds, bell peppers, parsley and dill.

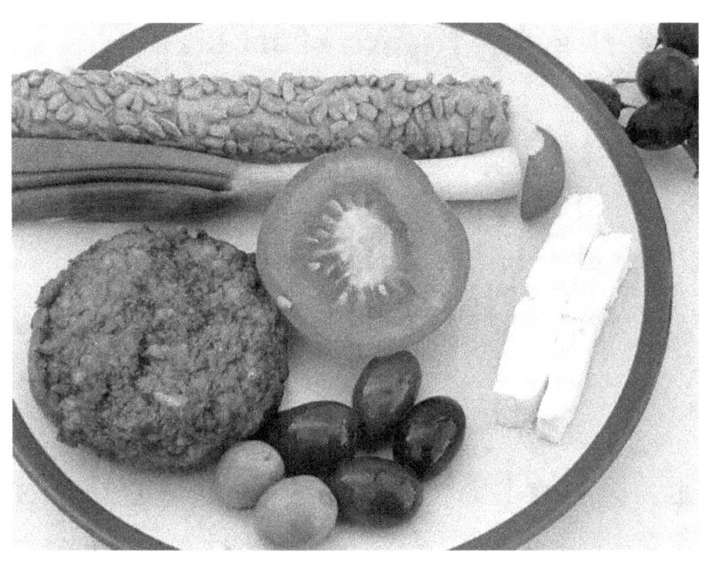

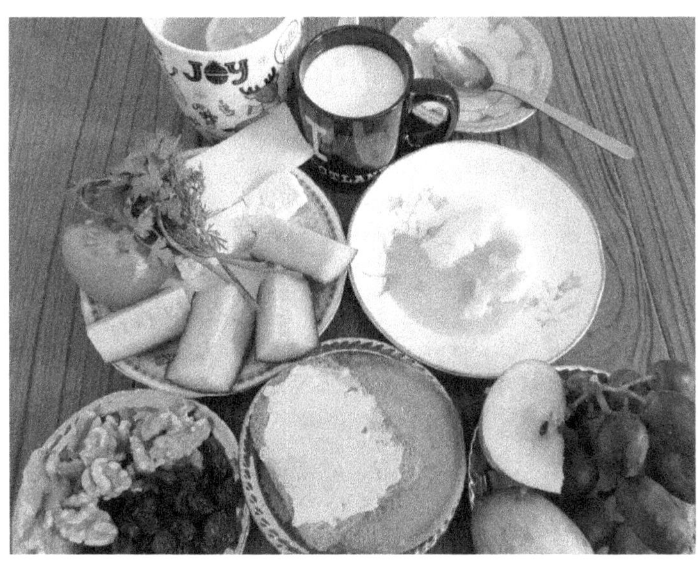

A few recipes for a healthy breakfast, because the day has to start strong

1. Breakfast recipe with cheese and bell pepper

White Greek cheese mixes well with dill, a drop of olive oil and sesame and / or sunflower seeds. The feta cheese also goes very well. So fill a green bell pepper with this mixture. Cut horizontally so that round slices result. A boiled egg cut in two halves and bread with seeds complete this recipe. It is simple, tasty, good-looking, healthy and easy to prepare.

2.Breakfast recipe with egg, butter and marmalade

It is probably the simplest and most suitable recipe for breakfast. Boil the eggs in such a way that the yolk remains soft, juicy, grease the wholemeal bread with a little butter and jam. It goes perfectly with a tea slightly sweetened with honey and flavored with a slice of lemon.

3. Breakfast recipe with fried bread, boiled egg and fresh oranges

This is my favorite recipe. As you've probably already noticed, I chose to recommend the morning meals that included the boiled egg. Why are you proud? Because it is a healthy food, easy to prepare, tasty and full of nutrients. Soft boiled egg and fried bread on the stove over which a slice of butter is placed. Complete the breakfast with a glass of fresh oranges. These may be enough until the next meal.

4. Breakfast recipe with Greek yogurt, honey and whole grains

I have chosen to offer you the simplest and healthiest recipes that anyone can prepare. Mix Greek yogurt with a little honey and whole grains. Eat a banana as a "dessert". But do not forget that the body needs exercise in addition to food.

5. Breakfast recipe with milk, cheese and bell pepper

Warm, unsweetened milk, slices of cheese and red bell pepper. Add a wholemeal bun and a nectarine / apricot / peach. They can provide you with the necessary nutrients. In addition, this breakfast does not need to be cooked and is very tasty and quick to prepare.

6. Breakfast recipe with boiled egg and feta cheese

Cut the soft boiled egg into small pieces. Mix with feta cheese and a little olive oil. It is eaten with slices of bread with seeds and fresh cucumber. A fresh orange or even some dried fruit at the end will turn this meal into a delicacy. But don't forget to prepare the right portions.

7. Breakfast recipe with cheese, olives, meatballs and tomatoes

Sometimes I prepare this simple and nutritious recipe for breakfast. A meatball, half a tomato and a few slices of cheese. I add olives, radishes and green onions. Top with a stick of sunflower seeds. In the end I eat a few grapes.

These recipes are designed to cover the need for nutrients until lunch. Of course, they can be adapted to your needs and possibilities.
Each people has its own breakfast habits. Italians, for example, eat bread with butter and jam and drink fresh oranges. Romanians can eat like Italians, but they can also eat a heavy meal, consisting of eggs, cheese and various sausages. I noticed that the Scots eat beans and sausages in the morning.
These habits most likely come from the needs of each people. In Italy, where it is always hot, it is normal for people to eat lighter foods. In Scotland, because the weather is much colder, it is natural for people to need more consistent food.

The food you eat must be adapted to your needs. If you are an active person, it is normal to eat more. If you live in a cold area of the earth, you will also need more food.

It is important not to eat until you can no longer get up from the table and be sure to exercise after eating. These are the most important elements in the process of eliminating extra pounds.

Final tips and tricks

- If you are an extroverted person, tell everyone that you are just trying a new (and yet so old) way to lose weight. Tell them about everything you do, because it is possible that this will help others who are facing the same problem. This will help you too, because it will motivate you to move on when you find it difficult, to be able to prove to others that you are a determined person, a strong character.
- If you are an introvert, it is probably better if you do not tell anyone until the results begin to be seen.
- Avoid fried foods.

- Avoid thinking about food all the time. Instead, choose to spend your time walking or enjoying your hobbies.
- Always drink a glass of water before a meal. This will help you feel full faster, which means you will eat less without feeling hungry.
- If you still feel the need to eat something between meals, especially in the first period, until your body adapts to change, choose to eat a fruit, not chocolate or pastries.
- If your health allows, drink a cup of coffee daily. Coffee can play an important role in digestion.
- Try to always have a good quality sleep. For this you need a dark and cool room, well ventilated, clean bed linen, a walk and not to drink too much fluid before bed (especially alcohol), because the bladder will demand its rights.
- Have full confidence that you will succeed. Even if you don't realize it yet, I knew from the moment you bought this book that you can fulfill your dream, that you will be able to lose weight effortlessly, that you will be beautiful and happy, what I wish you with all my heart!

Your feedback is very important to me.

In order for my message to reach as many people who are going through the same situation and fighting for the same goal,

I need your support.

If my book is useful to you, I will ask you to mention this in a review on the website where you bought it.

Thank you and I hope from the bottom of my heart that you will be satisfied too!

For any questions, advice or information in addition to what I wrote in the book, I am at your disposal whenever you need. Do not hesitate to contact me. I would be happy to talk and find out how you are doing and if you need support.

Contact details:

- sas.vienela@yahoo.com
- https://www.goodreads.com/author/show/21532693.Vienela_Sas
- https://www.amazon.co.uk/Vienela-Sas/e/B092MDGQW1
- https://www.facebook.com/sas.vienela/

Thank you! Stay safe!

www.ingramcontent.com/pod-product-compliance
Lightning Source LLC
Chambersburg PA
CBHW061546250726

48657CB00006B/2326